Plant-Based Superheroes

Incredible tales of Emergency Animal Rescues & Superheroes

Created by:

Shelly Fitzpatrick

FREE copies of this book are available to Children's Hospitals, Charities, and Women & Children's Shelters. You can email the author for requests or donations shellyfitzpatrickauthor@gmail.com

Copyright © 2020 Plant-Based Superheroes

All rights reserved. May not be copied without permission.

Published by: Empowering Kids Books and Fitzpatrick Rescue

Author: Shelly Fitzpatrick

Http://www.PlantbasedSuperheroes.com

Http://www.ShellyFitzpatrick.com

Illustrator: JB Mann

ISBN# 978-0-578-64650-3

ADVENTURES

1. Rescuing Baby Rio – the little turkey.

2. Hold on! It's a wild ride adventure with waterfalls!

3. Splashing into the Thank You, Sanctuary!

4. Romping Rascal, your red-carpet adventure tour guide.

5. Making Friends with Magic, Milo Mc Bark-A lot.

6. Meeting Baaashful the shy lamb and showing superhero kindness.

7. Bumping into Blurry Bobo, the blurred vision soccer playing dog.

ADVENTURES Continued:

8. Laughing with Comedian, Chili the Chicken and learning the real deal.

9. Partying with Pokey the pig, and hearing about his superhero rescue story.

10. Wakeboarding Wiggles, making waves.

11. Rascal's riveting emergency rescue tale.

12. Superhero powers you'll always have.

ADVENTURE #1. RESCUING BABY RIO, THE LITTLE TURKEY.

"Hurry come here! Can you hold her for a second?" Sounds the rescuer, who is a tall man with a kind face. He steps out of the truck he just raced down the driveway, and hands a small bird to Nate.

"I've got to get that box by the shed and a soft towel to put her in, so she feels safe." Says the rescuer.

Up until a minute ago, Nate was having a great time swinging back and forth on an old black tire swing. He was working hard to see how high he could get before jumping off to the ground.

Nate just watched the rescuer (his uncle, Quinn) drive hurriedly onto the remote sanctuary property while closing the wooden gate behind him. The dust from the truck having raced down the long dirt driveway is still flying all around and making circular swirls in the air. "Achoo" Nate sneezes from the dust.

Nate holds the tiny, newly feathered baby bird gently, as she nestles into his arms. The rescuer looks at Nate and tells him how he just rescued this baby turkey, and she needs their help now.

He explains to Nate that the little bird will be uncertain and unsure of them, until she settles in and realizes that she will be protected and safe at the sanctuary.

The rescuer picks back up the tiny, brown baby bird from Nate and gently places her in the box. The baby bird snuggles into the soft white towel and stretches her wings out, then brings them back in.

Nate looks precariously into the box with one funny raised eyebrow (that always makes people laugh.) "Will she fly away?" Nate asks. But the baby bird can't because she is only two weeks old.

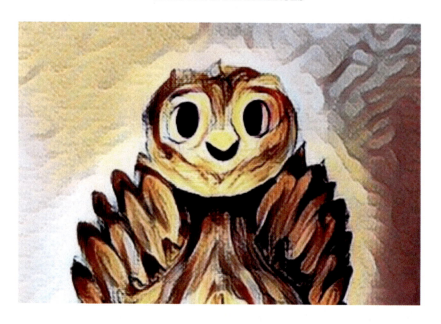

Nate scratches his head and continues looking curiously at the baby bird.

While bringing his hand to his face, the rescuer thinks about the best way to explain to Nate (his 8-year-old nephew, who is visiting for the summer) "why" this baby turkey needed to be rescued in the first place- as he knows the question is coming.

"But why did you rescue this bird, Uncle Quinn?" Nate surely asks.

The rescuer smiles and shakes his head up and down, knowing it was the exact question he was expecting from Nate.

Lately, Nate has been asking a lot of the "But why this?" "But why that?" questions.

The rescuer ponders how to explain to Nate the difficult realities in the world that people like him, and others are trying to change.

"Can we pleaaaaase give her a name?" Nate suddenly begs.

"I bet I can come up with a terrific name that suits her best!"

What do you think about Snuggles, the baby bird?

Or maybe Shiloh, the shy bird? No, I've got it, Baby Sky, the Fly Bird!

Wait, I really have it now...

Let's name her... Baby Rio! Yes, that's it. May we name her Baby Rio?"

The rescuer smiles widely and welcomes the sweet name Nate just came up with for the baby turkey.

The rescuer knows there is always a magical and special bond between a kid and an animal when the kid gets to name their new friend.

ADVENTURE #2. HOLD ON! IT'S A WILD RIDE ADVENTURE WITH WATERFALLS!

"I can't believe how exciting this is! I didn't sleep a wink last night." Expressed Kaia, (a strong, brave, and caring girl, with long blond hair) who is standing by the giant yellow and black school bus. Kaia continues, "I even dreamt about what it must be like at the Thank You, Sanctuary."

"I was told it is an amazingly fun place with special activities for kids. With tons of interesting animals to see, and we can even play with them. I also heard it is a 100% safe and fully protected sanctuary for rescued animals." Says a kid on the bus.

"My teacher mentioned something about being a Vegetable-tarian or whatever, and we would learn valuable lessons about why we shouldn't eat animals." Shares Jake (a happy-go-lucky kid who always wears his favorite blue baseball hat.)

One of the other school kids (who is a beautiful dark complexion girl, wearing a pink "Kindness Rules") shirt says, "Yeah, the school bus driver told me this is a magical bus and the only school bus in the entire world that can bring kids to the Sanctuary."

As the kids are boarding and sitting down on the magical school bus, they begin to feel the tires becoming super inflated.

They look outside the windows and see the tires inflating and beginning to look like giant chocolate doughnuts.

The kids all laugh out loud and share their excitement for what they are about to experience today.

The bus suddenly lifts up and takes off. It feels like they are riding on a cloud in the air- like a soft, cushy, cloud mobile. The kids continue to smile and laugh.

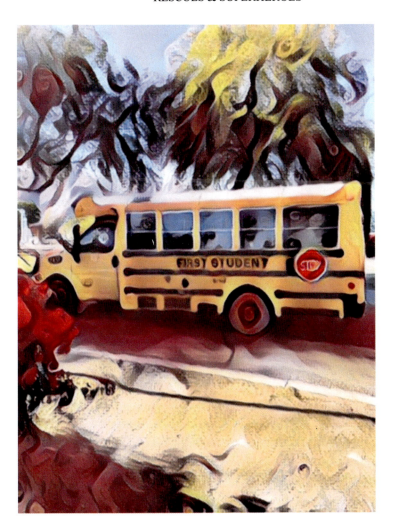

As the school bus is floating along with the cloud lined highways and curvy roads, it ascends mountains and rocky hills. The laughing continues, as the kids are all slowly bouncing up and down in their seats.

The bus driver (a caring and funny older woman with white hair, and large green glasses) looks in her rear-view mirror and laughs out loud as she catches some of the kids in mid-air! It looks like the kids are moving in slow motion.

Then the roaring sound of splashing water is heard. They begin to approach massive, light blue waterfalls that are spraying water everywhere!

The kids on the bus shout, "Check out those huge waterfalls! Look out! We are going to get wet!" The water starts spraying into the bus and splattering on the kids as they pass the waterfalls.

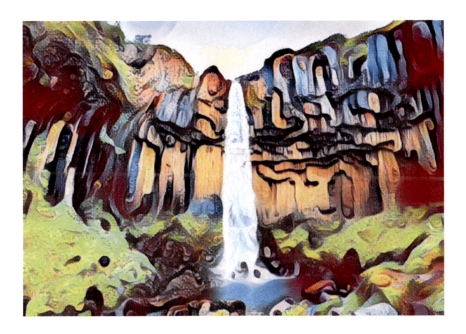

"This is hilarious!" "We are totally getting drenched!" Shouts the kids.

Water begins filling up the black lined floor of the school bus, and the kid's shoes get wet.

Jake and Kaia wipe the water from their sunglasses. It looks like windshield wipers on the front window of a car during a rainstorm.

ADVENTURE #3. SPLASHING INTO THE THANK YOU SANCTUARY.

"We did it!" "We have finally arrived!", alerts the cheerful school bus driver to the kids. After a fun and exhilarating school bus adventure, they have finally pulled up to the special main gate in front of the private, Thank You, Sanctuary.

Nate, who is still with his uncle caring for the bird (and waiting on hearing the story of her rescue), suddenly hears a loud sound of screeching brakes. Nate turns around and blurts out, "Look, there is a school bus at your gate!"

The rescuer appreciates the brief pause from having to explain the details of the turkey ranch, where Baby Rio was rescued.

"Yes, Nate. I invited some school kids to visit our special sanctuary today to play with the animals and learn the sanctuary's secrets." He tells Nate that he is old enough now to get answers to all of those "But Why?" questions about the sanctuary he so often asks.

Nate takes a deep breath and lets out a loud "gulp" from his throat. Nate ponders what secrets will be divulged today.

Meanwhile, the kids can barely contain their enthusiasm and can't wait to exit the school bus!

As the bus driver pulls the large handle, the doors slowly squeak open, the kids jump out and begin running down a steep hill.

With so much excitement built up, Jake trips over his untied shoelaces. He falls and accidentally knocks down Kaia in the process. They both begin falling and rolling down the hill.

They look like a burrito covered in grass, like out of a comedy movie!

Then "swoosh!" They roll and splash right into a large, bright blue shimmering swimming pool. They totally go underwater and get submerged! As they rise back up from the water and wipe their eyes, they see a gray dog standing and surfing on an orange boogie board in the pool. They can't believe it!

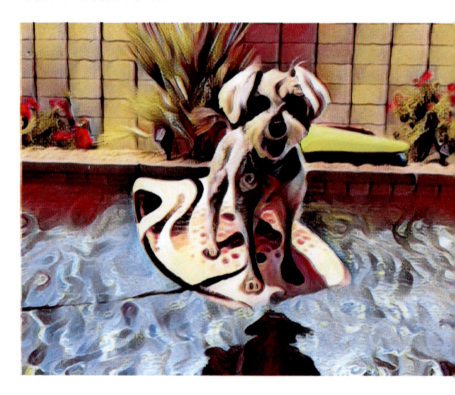

They see hundreds of animals all playing in and around the pool while laughing uncontrollably at the kids! The ducks are swimming over to ensure the kids are ok from their fall.

Jake and Kaia hear music, birds singing, and lots of laughing. They see all kinds of cool-looking animals. Ducks and geese are swimming and playing in the pool. There are even cute, pink pigs swimming in the water, with birds on their heads.

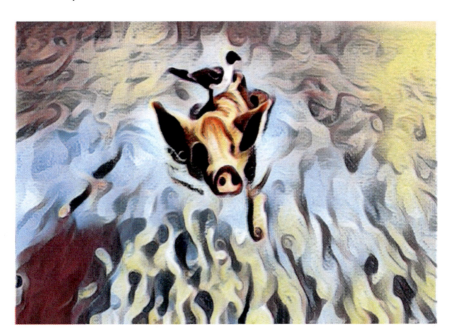

Water fountains are shooting water 1000 feet high up in the air, and the ducks are goofing around in it. Music is playing to the sound of water as it squirts up and drops back down to the musical beats.

The ducks are laughing while lying on their backs floating on flamingo, penguin, and big white and rainbow unicorn rafts. They mimic the waterfall and begin shooting water out of their mouths, high up into the sky.

As the ducks spray the water up, it drops back down on them, which makes them laugh even more!

Nate and his uncle Quinn are still laughing at having watched the spectacle of the kids rolling down the hill and splashing into the pool.

The rescuer calls out to the kids, "Hey, I'm sure glad you kids can swim! Please grab those orange towels on the brown lounge chairs and come over here."

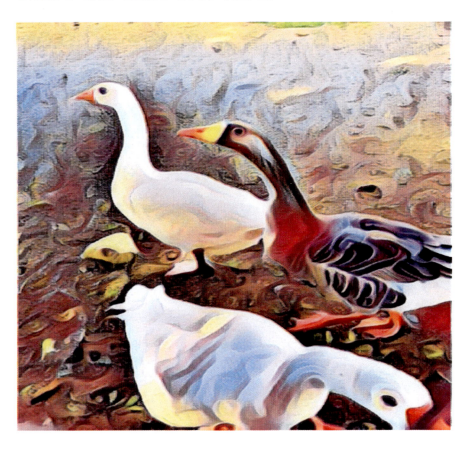

Kaia and Jake smile as they walk and squish with each step and take their soaked selves over to the rescuer, Nate, and where the other kids who stayed dry gathered.

"Hello kids, I'm Quinn, and I run the Thank You Sanctuary, and this is my nephew Nate. He spends his summers here with me, and the animals that I have rescued."

I was just about to tell Nate the story behind the rescue of this baby bird. Would you all like to hear it?"

Nate, being so curious lately, excitedly and immediately sits down, crosses his legs, and rests his chin on top of his hands and says, "Yes, please tell me, because I was about to ask you that question."

The kids all agree and sit down next to Quinn, waiting to hear the intriguing tale. "Today, we are going to share the real stories of rescue with you," shares Quinn.

Nate lifts that one eyebrow again and asks, "What do you mean, "WE?" As the rescuer and Nate have been the only humans at the sanctuary EVER, until the school bus arrived.

"Hold on little buddy, and I will get to that." Uncle Quinn (the rescuer) begins explaining to Nate and the kids who just arrived, the conditions thousands of turkeys were living in at the ranch where Baby Rio had just been rescued.

He takes a deep breath and shares what he saw during the rescue. As he does, he feels the droplets of tears beginning to form and build up in his eyes. He desperately tries to keep those tears from falling while explaining the rescue. He begins to tell the kids how the conditions at the turkey ranch were horrible.

He explains, "There were thousands of turkeys living in cramped, filthy cages. During all of the chaos, I was able to swoop in and rescue this little turkey, and Nate just named her, Baby Rio."

"She was very dependent on her mommy, (as all babies are,) but her mommy and many other turkeys were suddenly and abruptly taken away." Shares Quinn.

"But I was able to save Baby Rio. And starting today, we are going to rehabilitate her (that means to make her better) and help her feel safe and secure again."

Kaia chime's in, "Wow, that is great you saved her!" Nate chimes in, "But why did they take all of those other turkeys, and where did they take them, Uncle Quinn?"

Then an unfamiliar voice from a short distance away says, "Whoa!" "We have company today?"

The kids all look around confusingly to see who said that, as it certainly didn't come from their group.

ADVENTURE #4. ROMPING RASCAL, YOUR RED-CARPET ADVENTURE TOUR GUIDE.

Then out from a bright and shiny red barn, a ton of fluffy and puffy animals start pouring out and talking.

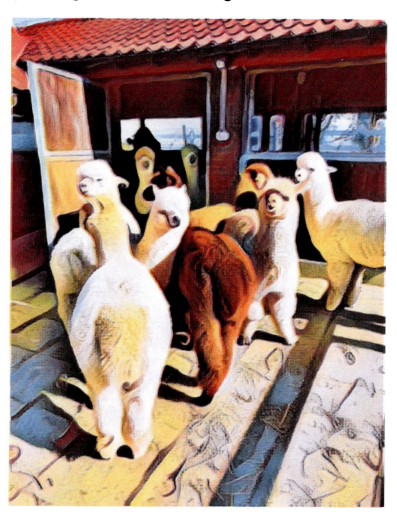

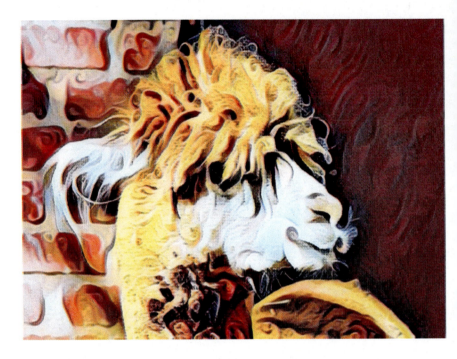

One in particular is a curiously, funny-looking animal. A real loaf of a character, with a furry white and tan coat, a brown mohawk, and protruding teeth sticking out.

It has goofy-looking eyeballs and the biggest smile on its face! Quinn announces, "Kids, this is Rascal. Good to see you, Rascal! How are you doing today, my friend?" Asks Quinn.

"I'm doing great today! I was playing with my friends when we heard all the splashing coming from the pool, and it interrupted our checkers game. But it's ok, its no-prob-Llama. (Ha ha ha!) Llamas are cool too. But you know me, I'm not a Llama, I'm an Alpaca!" Shares Rascal.

"Alpacas like me are smaller, and our teeth stick out far and wide. This is why people always smile and laugh when they see us. And I say hey, if that makes people happy then giddy up! That's fine with me." Continues Rascal.

Rascal continues to educate the kids. "Alpacas are herd animals, and that means we love to be around other animals! Being a part of a pack makes us super happy! I especially like to have fun, be silly, and spend time with my friends."

"Hey, will y'all kids be my new friends?" Asks Rascal.

Nate and the school kids are flabbergasted and staring in amazement and wonderment.

Their mouths are wide open and almost hitting the floor. Not to mention, their eyes are as big as bowling balls, as no one has ever heard an animal speak before!

A stunned and bewildered Jake stutters the words, "Wa, Wh, wait, wait a minute... You can talk?"

"Heck Yeah, I sure can!" trumpets Rascal. "Come here. I'll let you in on a little secret." The kids cautiously, (yet excitedly) approach and lean into Rascal. "Yeah, what?" Says the kids. As they anticipatedly wait to hear the secret.

"While you are at the Thank You, Sanctuary, you will be able to understand what we are saying, BUT ONLY HERE."

"Today I will teach you how to understand animals, so y'all can help them when they need it. Sort of like being an animal whisperer, like that guy on tv with dogs.

Rascal says, "Right now, I dub ye, The Alpaca Whisperers." "Ha Ha Ha!" Everyone laughs.

The rescuer smiles and pats Rascal on his fluffy, puffy, head. He tells the kids they are in good hands with Rascal today, and that Rascal will show them around the sanctuary and introduce them to the other animals. Rascal obliges and asks the kids, "So, what are your names?"

"Rascal, it's me, Nate. You know me. I visit you every summer. I never knew you could speak! My Uncle said I was old enough, now that I'm 8, to learn the truth about animals and the secrets of the sanctuary."

Rascal says, "Of course, I know you, Nate!" I love it when you visit us each summer!"

"Uh, Hi Rascal. I'm Kaia, and I'm super excited to meet you and see this special place. But, I'm totally shocked that you can talk." Then the rest of the kids all introduce themselves.

"And last but not least, I'm Jake! You look super cool, Rascal! We will gladly be your friends!" "Great! It is very nice to meet you all. Says Rascal. "You will totally dig this place. Bravery, kindness, and friendships flourish here, at the Thank You, Sanctuary."

"How about I take you around to meet my friends? I guarantee you will love them, and they will love you." Says Rascal.

"Ok, that's awesome!" says the kids. Nate picks up the box that Baby Rio is in, so she can be carried around with them today.

"It will be great for her to meet the other animals here. Let's all help her feel safe and loved today." Nate proudly shares.

Baby Rio has her face tucked in under one wing. She pokes one white and black eyeball out, so she can assess the situation. She is still unsure of what's going on, as she has been through a lot lately.

Kaia reaches in the box and gives baby Rio a gentle, reassuring pet on her wing. "It's going to be better now, you will see. You are safe here. This place seems pretty amazing!" Says Kaia.

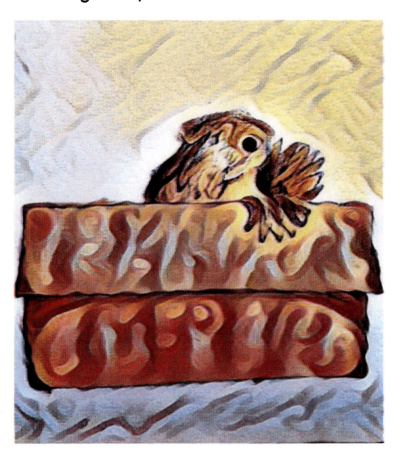

ADVENTURE #5. MAKING FRIENDS WITH MAGIC, MILO MC BARK A LOT.

Rascal begins showing the kids around the sanctuary as she grazes the grass, eating up green grass chunks along the way.

When surprisingly, a dog comes up from behind and wraps his paws around Rascal's eyes and says, "Guess who?"

Rascal lifts her shoulders in excitement, "I know that voice! That's the voice of my best friend, Milo." The dog drops his paws around Rascal's eyes, and Rascal turns around and says, "Hey kids, I'd like to introduce you all to Milo Mc'*Bark-A lot.*"

Milo's tail is wagging very quickly side-to-side. His bright white, furry coat and ears are bouncing up and down, while he is jumping around and barking non-stop with excitement.

"Check out Milo! He is a very sharp dresser. He always wears his finest tuxedo when he meets new friends." Says Rascal.

"Milo was rescued from the streets, where someone abandoned him. He had no food, no shelter, and no clean clothes. His fur was so bad that it turned into dreadlocks. And I'm not talking about the cool Rastafarian kind. But look at him now, since he's been saved! He looks like a prince with a million bucks! He is the kindest soul I know." Shares Rascal.

Milo Mc'Bark-A lot greets each kid with paw high-fives and paw fist-bumps. Milo asks, "Who do we have here in this box that you are carrying?"

"This is Baby Rio," Kaia says. "Nate's uncle told us about how she was just rescued. We are helping to take care of her right now and make her feel safe."

Milo looks in the box, "It's my distinguished pleasure to meet you, Baby Rio."

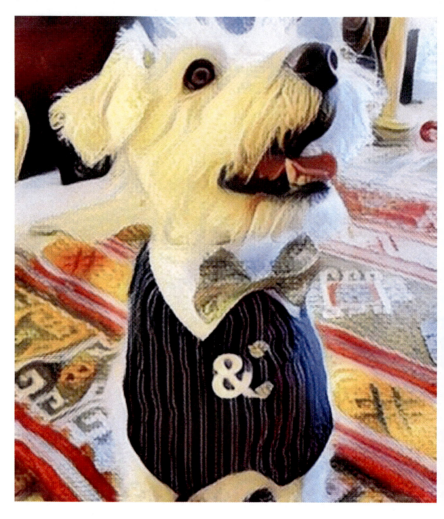

Rio looks up at Milo and gives a shy, side smile. She can't help but smile when she sees Milo, as she can tell he is a kind-hearted dog.

Milo asks the kids, "Do you have dogs like me in your family?"

"Yeah, I do! I have two at home, and they are my best friends. They love to play with toys and chase balls and Frisbee's. They love to sleep at my feet every night. They are *supposed* to sleep in their fluffy, deluxe pet beds, but that never happens." chuckles Jake.

Kaia adds, "I have a dog too. She is tiny, and when she sleeps, she sprawls out all over my entire bed! It's like she becomes 200 feet long. I'm always waking up in the morning like a contortionist pretzel." Hahaha! Everyone laughs!

"Here, check out this photo of her. She loves it when I dress her up, take snap chat photos, and post them on my social media sites. Isn't she cool looking with her tight shades on! Her name is AJ." Shares Kaia.

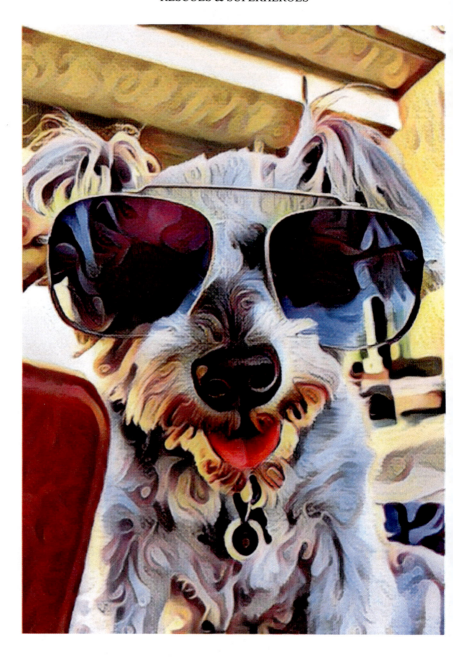

While the kids are huddled around Kaia, looking at pictures of her dog AJ, Rascal slips away for a minute. She heads over to a small shed, where there is a silver refrigerator inside.

On the fridge door, there are red flashing words on it that read, "Don't Drink Me." Rascal naturally grabs a few bottles from the refrigerator and darts back over to the kids.

"Would y'all like to try a magical potion that Milo created?" Rascal holds the bottles and whirls them teasingly around the kids, with a prankster's gleam in her eyes.

"This magical potion will make your spoken words come out like a dog's bark." Shares Rascal. Jake immediately grabs the bottle from Rascal and shouts, "Bottoms up!"

He guzzles the liquid (gulp, gulp, gulp,) then takes a breath and begins to speak. "Ruff, Ruff, Ruff. Woof, Woof, Woof! Bow, Wow, Wow!"

The kid's necks go backward, and their eyes practically pop out of their sockets as they howl in laughter!

"Jake, you are barking like a dog!" Says Kaia. Rascal and Milo are holding their bellies and rolling on the floor in laughter!

"Don't worry, it wears off after 90 seconds." Shares Rascal.

"Ruff, ruff, ruff, bark, bark, bark... Hello?" Jake gets his regular words back and asks, "What on earth was that stuff? That's wild! It made me bark like a dog. I kept asking if you understood me, but I don't think you did."

Nate asks Rascal, "Is that what it's like when you try to speak to people outside of the sanctuary?" Rascal nods and says, "Yep! Animals feel pretty scared and alone when they can't tell people what they are thinking and how they are feeling.

Hopefully, you kids are beginning to get what it's like for us animals."

Milo begins running in circles around the kids. "Follow me, follow me, follow me! I will take you to a special place where we can hang out with some of our interesting friends. You won't believe your eyes and ears when you meet them! Come on, follow me!"

ADVENTURE #6. MEETING BAAASHFUL, THE SHY LAMB AND SHOWING SUPERHERO KINDENESS.

Everyone starts skipping and meandering across the finely cut grass, and they arrive at a brown building with a sign above that reads, "Welcome to the *Laughing Lamb Lounge. Where all your worries leave, and the laughter lingers.*"

Rascal leads them inside the very crowded lounge. As they maneuver their way through the lambs in the lounge, they realize it is too crowded in there for them. It sure looks like a lot fun though. The lambs are laughing, talking, drinking juice, and playing cards. But Nate looks out a window and can see what looks like a baby lamb in the distance, who is not participating in the fun.

Nate motions to Rascal and the other kids to leave the lounge, so they can get a better look and see what's going on with the baby lamb outside. They make their way out by turning sideways left, then sideways right, through all the lambs, and exit the Laughing Lamb Lounge.

They stride across the field and see a young, white lamb in baby blue pajamas. "I thought that might be you." Says Rascal. "How are you doing today, BaaaShful?"

BaaaShful looks at Rascal and the kids and gives a little smile and shrugs her fluffy shoulders. "I'm doing better now that you came over to say hi to me."

Rascal explains to the kids that BaaaShful is new to the sanctuary, and she is still a bit timid and shy.

Things were rough for her when she was growing up, but she is safe now. Everyone is helping her get better each and every day.

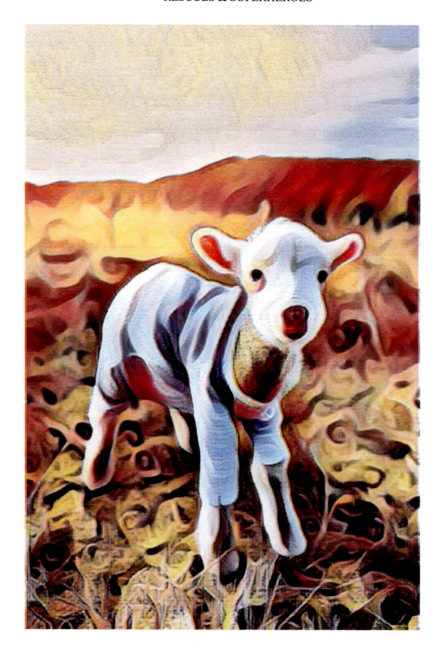

Rascal explains to the kids how there is good and bad in the world.

She tells the kids how BaaaShful had a very difficult start to life, but then she got rescued and brought to the sanctuary for her safety.

Rascal shares with the kids to be friendly when they meet someone shy, as it could be they are nervous, insecure, or had something bad happen to them. Be brave and say "Hello" to the shy ones. They are the ones who need it the most!" Says Rascal.

She continues, "Kids, you can help animals like BaaaShful and Baby Rio by making this world really great for animals. Did you know that you have superpowers that can help animals?" Milo chimes in, "Yeah, did you know that? It's so cool!"

Jake immediately opens his mouth, "I've never heard of kids having real-life superpowers. I thought that was just in the movies."

"Wait, we do?" Asks Kaia and the other kids.

Rascal replies, "You sure do! All kids have superpowers, but not all kids know how to activate and use them."

"You are very special, because **kids** are the **chosen ones** to **protect animals**."

"By starting now, when you are young, you can activate this extraordinary power inside of you and use it throughout your lifetime. Your superpowers can help to change bad things to good." Explains Rascal. He then asks the kids,

"Can you say, *I can change bad things to good?*"

Kids shout out, "I can change bad things to good!"

"Great!" "Wow, I'm impressed!" Says Rascal

Then BaaaShful, with a big, evolving smile on her face says, "Thank you! That is very kind of you kids"

Rascal thanks BaaaShful for sharing some of her time with the kids and says goodbye.

However, just as everyone is saying their goodbyes and about to leave, a black and white soccer ball goes whizzing by Nate's face at the speed of light, and almost knocks him down. "What? What was that?" Asks Nate.

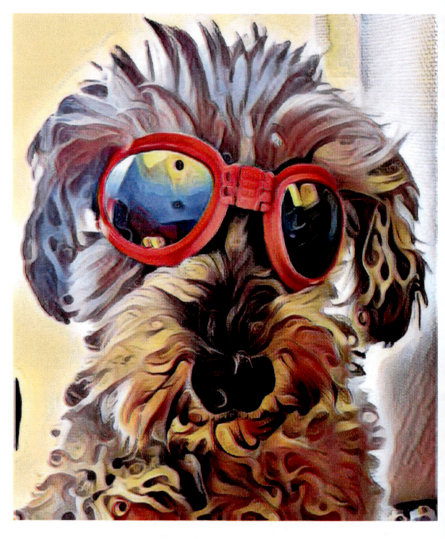

Its Bobo, the blurred vision, red goggles wearing, soccer-playing dog!

ADVENTURE #7. LOOK OUT, IT'S BOBO THE BLURRED VISION SOCCER-PLAYING DOG

Rascal knew Bobo would be following shortly behind the soccer ball which came catapulting out of the sky and nearly flattened Nate to the ground! Bobo loves to play soccer, but she has serious vision problems, so you usually have to duck and dodge flying soccer balls that she kicks.

And wouldn't you know it, just like clockwork, a white and grey, red prescription goggled wearing dog, comes running up to Nate and the kids. "Have you seen my soccer ball?" Inquires the confused, shaggy dog with her tongue sticking out.

"Yeah, I see it, hang on." Rascal trots over to the soccer ball and kicks the ball back to Bobo. "Kids come on. Let's run with Bobo back to the soccer field and play." Suggests Rascal.

Milo and the kids follow Rascal and Bobo to the soccer field. As they approach the goal, Bobo shoots, she scores, oops... Nope!

Instead, Bobo kicks the soccer ball smack dab into the goalie pole, and the soccer ball goes flying backwards. "Duck!" screams out, Rascal. The ball just misses Kaia's face this time, and everyone is laughing.

Bobo thinks she scored a goal, so everyone cheers to make her feel good. "How do you like my tight soccer skills?" Asks a panting and out of breath Bobo. Nate smiles and chuckles under his breath, "Uh, you play like a pro, Bobo!" Bobo replies, "Thanks Nate, I certainly have fun playing soccer! Hey, I'm getting kind of hungry now, would you mind pouring some food into my bowl?"

Kaia agrees to pour Bobo's food. "Sure, that sounds like fun!" Rascals shows Kaia where the food is, and she begins to pour the food into Bobo's bowl.

Bobo graciously responds. "Thank you so much! You know everyone gets hungry right? And eating is very important. Did you know that "what" you eat matters?" Bobo, now sounding like a non-confused, highly intelligent dog declares.

While giving Bobo a notoriously dubious look, Nate asks, "But why?" Nate loves the opportunity to ask his famous ("but why questions.")

"Well, food can give you energy, like what we have while playing soccer. It can also make you healthy or unhealthy, and it can hurt you (and us animals,) depending upon the kind of food you eat." Bobo shares.

Nate decides to probe even further and asks, "So what kind of food do you eat?" Bobo tilts her head to the side, motioning towards her bowl, which has food in it. "Take a look. It is all plant-based dog food." Says Bobo.

Then Rascal chimes in, "Check out the bucket on the ground for us alpacas, too." The kids start to walk over, but this time Kaia jumps ahead of Jake and begins running over to the bucket.

She looks down into the bucket and sees piles of small, firm, green macaroni looking noodles and asks, "What is this stuff, Rascal?"

Rascal answers, "Those are my yummy pellets, and us Alpaca's are called Herbivores. Big word, I know! It's hard for us to pronounce it too."

"I say it like this, Herb-I-Vores. Ha ha ha."

"These pellets keep us healthy and strong, and no animals are harmed to make our food. Isn't that great! "Will you feed me too? I'm starved from all of the soccer playing!"

Kaia digs her hand into the bucket and

pulls up a large pile of green pellets. As she places her hand just below Rascal's mouth to begin feeding her, Bobo blindly sticks her mouth in between the two, and begins chomping up and devouring the pellets in a flurried rush.

"Munch, munch, munch." Bobo's face is all-up in the pellets, and they begin flying everywhere as she eats. Some pellets get into Bobo's mouth and others go launching into the air, like a helicopter propeller is spreading them! "Ping, ting, bong!" The pellets go flying and hit the shed. All the kids are laughing uncontrollably.

As she continues to eat, pellets start hitting Kaia, Jake, Nate, and Milo in the face, and they all start cracking up.

Bobo has a huge smile on her face, and everyone around is laughing at the sight of Bobo unintentionally eating Rascal's food.

After 15 minutes of munch, munch, munch,

and propelling pellets, a really loud "BURP!" comes out from Bobo's mouth. "Oops, excuse me. Hahaha! I think I am pretty full now. Thank you for feeding me." Says Bobo. The kids all laugh, as that was Rascal's food Bobo was eating!

Want to run around and play another game of soccer with Bobo?" Asks a kind, hungry Rascal. The kids all willfully smile and trot back out onto the grass soccer field. But Kaia heads back to the bucket and grabs another handful of pellets and brings them to Rascal. "Here you go, Rascal. I bet you are still hungry. You sure are a nice alpaca who cares about others." Says Kaia.

The kids to start kicking the ball to one another, shooting goals, (and of course,) dodging the flying soccer balls being kicked by Bobo. Nate yells out, "Duck!" as another ball goes flying past Milo's head this time. "Hey, what's that sound I hear?" Asks Jake.

ADVENTURE #8. LAUGHING WITH COMEDIAN, CHILLI THE CHICKEN AND LEARNING THE REAL DEAL

Jake hears the sound of laughter in the distance and wonders what's so funny? Nate's left eyebrow lifts up again, as he has a question that needs to be answered. "May we go see where all that laughter is coming from? Asks Nate.

"You bet! Let's say goodbye to Bobo and go over there so we can find out." Says Rascal.

Bobo and the kids thank one another and say their goodbyes. Rascal tells Bobo she will see her later, then nudges the kids to run quickly towards the sound of all that laughter.

As they run through the grassy field, they see signs that read, "Get Your Laugh On, Comedy Special." They arrive and see a bunch of chickens all huddled in a circle.

"Stop it, I can't breathe!" "She is so funny!" The chickens say as they are leaning on one another, holding their stomachs and laughing.

The kids manage to get to the center of the circle where they see a chicken holding an old nostalgic, shiny silver microphone and telling hilariously funny jokes to the chicken crowd.

After the comedian finishes the joke, Rascal approaches the swanky looking comedian and says, "I'd like to introduce you, kids, to the very funny comedian, "Chilli, The Chicken."

"Yep, even her name is funny!"

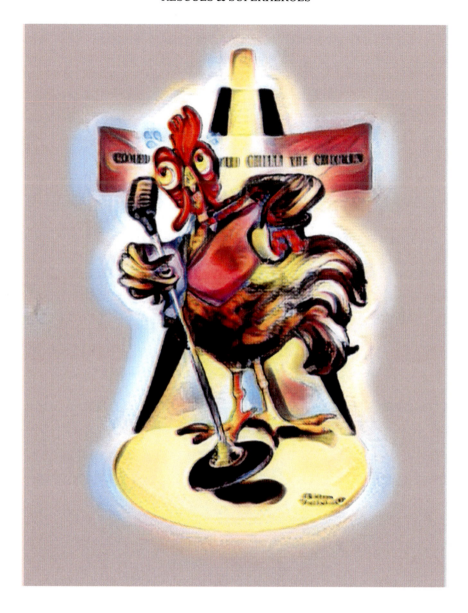

Chilli says in a high-pitched voice, "Hi kids, it's great to meet you!

Want to hear a joke?"

Kids shout, "Yes!"

Chilli grabs hold of the silver microphone, leans it to the side and asks:

"Do you know why the chicken crossed the playground?"

(Slight pause)

"To get to the other S L I D E!"

"Hahahaha!"

The kids laugh out loud! Then a sound comes out from the box below. ("Ha Ha!")

Everyone looks down and sees baby Rio has a huge glowing smile on her face and she is cracking up!

Chilli smiles lovingly, as she can tell Baby Rio was recently rescued, so this makes Chilli very happy, knowing she helped to make her laugh.

Ding-dong, ding-dong, ding-doooonnnngggg. A clock on the barn wall begins ringing. "It's lunchtime, it's lunchtime!" The chickens announce into the microphone with a little tap dance in unison.

"You just caught me at the end of my set. I'm starved! Are you kids hungry? Have you had lunch yet?" Chili grabs some brown paper lunch bags and asks the kids, "Would like to share my delicious plant-based sandwiches and tacos?"

"Whoa, thanks, but isn't plant-based food just for animals? Do you have any turkey sandwiches, since it is almost Thanksgiving?" Asks Jake.

"Do you have any chicken nuggets?" Asks Kaia. I always eat those when I go to...

Chilli screeches out in a high pitch shriek!!! "Eeeeeekkkk!!" "Yikes!" "You want... What?" Then a flurry of chicken feet is heard running away from the kids. All the chickens are now hiding behind some trees- and baby Rio's box begins moving backwards.

Kaia stares at Chilli with a startled and confused look on her face. Then a wave of understanding and a slight embarrassment comes over her.

"Wait... YOU are a chicken. Do you mean we eat animals like you? Is it the same thing?" Asks Kaia.

Chilli says, "Yes, that's Exact-A-Mundo, exactly correct. That's the real deal. Even when they label the food *"chicken"* and *"turkey,"* people still don't make the connection.

I'm glad you kid's just figured it out, and so quickly too, I might add!"

But Jake isn't convinced of this new-found knowledge and decides to slowly, inch-by-inch, take steps backwards and walks away from the group.

Nate says, "If we are here to be your friends and protectors, then we shouldn't eat turkeys or chicken's like you. I get it now!" He shouts!

Chili says, "Thanks, kids. That sure would mean a lot if you wouldn't eat us. Instead, you can use your superpowers to protect us, as we can't protect ourselves."

"Whoa! This is the second time today I have heard these superpowers mentioned? How do we get these superpowers?" Asks a very curious Kaia.

Chilli begins grinning ear to ear and explains, "Well kids, you EARN your superpowers when you protect animals and don't eat them. You are given superpowers of strength, courage, and bravery.

These are superpowers that all kids have inside of them, but not all kids know how to use them. So, the fact that you are willing to learn and use your superpowers to protect animals, that makes you very special! Remember, animals are 100% dependent upon YOU to protect them.

It's great to know you kids now understand a chicken nugget and chicken sandwich, are really chickens like me and my friends and inside of those meals."

Chilli asks the kids, "Do you know why Baby Rio is here?" The kids tell Chilli they heard she needed to be rescued, but they didn't get the full story yet.

"Well, Baby Rio was rescued because her parents and millions of other turkeys are taken away abruptly during a time called Thanksgiving.

It's odd because people are giving "thanks" on that day for many things, especially for their families, yet the turkeys are being "taken away" from their families, so people can eat them." Explains Chilli.

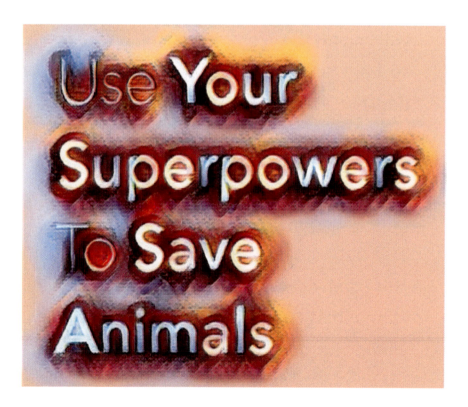

Baby Rio slowly peers up from inside the box, sniffs, and lets out a sad sigh, (as she witnessed what happened to her family and the other turkey families that day.)

Rascal adds, "I know some of this is a little heavy right now for you kids, but us animals really want you to know the truth."

Chilli nods her head in agreement.

"We believe if you are told the truth, you will make the right decisions going forward, to help save animals and protect your own health.

So, let's eat these yummy plant-based sandwiches that don't include animals." Suggests Rascal.

The kids start eating and chowing down on the sandwiches and love them! Kaia says, "They taste like our other sandwiches, just minus the animals. I love it!"

Jake's tummy is heard rumbling in the distance, so he begrudgingly decides to walk back to the group and give the plant-based food a try. While making a snarky face, he takes a small bite of a sandwich, (like a tiny mouse with a big piece of cheese.)

Then he takes a bigger bite, and all of a sudden, the whole sandwich is gone in one fail swoop! "Gulp!" "Wow, this is actually really good! I'm going to tell my friends and family about this food!" Thank you, Chilli!" Says Jake.

The kids finish their lunch and thank Chilli for the laughs, lessons and food.

Rascal adds, "Oh, and you won't believe who you are going to meet next!"

ADVENTURE #9. PARTYING WITH POKEY THE PIG, AND HEARING ABOUT HIS SUPERHERO RESCUE STORY.

The kids excitedly begin skipping along the grounds towards the next set of friends they will meet. As they are moving along kicking one leg forward and one leg back, they approach a big pink barn, with pink shiny strobe lights, flashing as far as the eye can see. They hear fun music and sounds coming from the barn. ♪♪♪♪

"Boom, Boom, Boom, Dance, Dance, Dance, Wee, Wee, Wee, Fun, Fun, Fun!" The crowd roars! There is always music, singing, and dancing at the pink, pig barn.

The kids open the big, bright, pink door and cascade in. Rascal points out a pig dancing on the black and white checkered dance floor. "That's my friend, Pokey. I bet he can teach us some cool dance moves today."

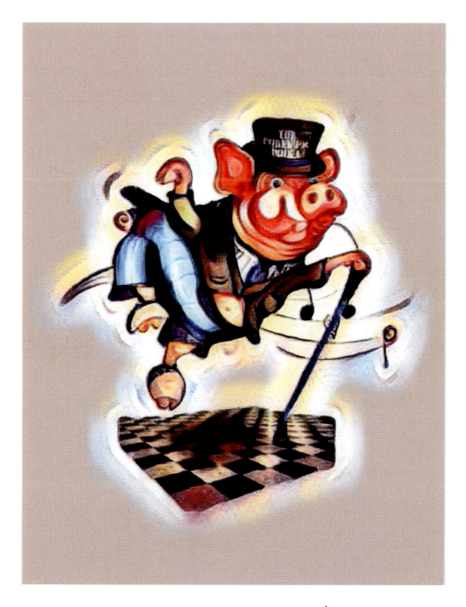

The pig shouts over the music, "Rascal, come join me on the dance floor and bring your friends."

They strut over to the dancing pig, who is wearing blue slacks, tuxedo tails, and a black gentleman's top hat. He is also surprisingly agile for a large pig.

"Hi Pokey, thanks for calling us over." Says Rascal. The kids all greet Pokey and begin dancing with him on the dance floor. "This is lots of fun!" Says Nate.

"Want to learn some cool dance moves?" Asks Pokey? The kids all smile, laugh, and absolutely agree to learn. Pokey begins teaching the kids the "Pig Jive dance" and the "Pig Twirly Turn dance," along with all the latest and coolest dance moves. Everyone is dancing, singing, and having an exhaustingly great time!

After 60 mins of non-stop dancing, Kaia decides to check in on Baby Rio. Much to her surprise, she sees the little turkey is moving her feet to the beat. Kaia gives Baby Rio a big smile and a hand-to-wing high five! "You're going to be okay, Baby Rio" Kaia says warmly.

The DJ announces there will be a brief break, and everyone falls down to the floor in laughter and sheer exhaustion. Pokey laughs and thanks the kids for dancing with him.

With everyone tired and all out of breath, Rascal suggests they go outside to get some fresh air. They leave the barn and walk outside to a table, which of course is pink and has sparkles all over it.

"I just love it here! I'm so thankful I was rescued and brought here." Shares Pokey. "Did you know I was once at a farm with many other pigs like me? Yep, we were all crammed and squished into tight spaces and cages. We couldn't even move around, and we realized it wasn't going to be any fun.

One night, we overheard a person saying they were intending on selling us and turning us into food, so people could eat us.

"Yikes!" Kaia responds. "What?" "Why you?" Pokey answers, "Well, they just don't care about animals."

"All animals are kept far away from the people who eat them, so they don't see us and can't hear our cries for help. If they did, I bet you a million dollars they wouldn't eat animals anymore." Declares Pokey.

"You know, most people actually LOVE animals, especially KIDS!" Shares Rascal.

"Yep, people just don't know the truth that it is "animals like us" on their food plates." Pokey continues, "But one incredible night, I was saved, and my life changed forever! There was a really nice woman with kids, who came in and rescued my little sister and me from that farm.

I learned those people are called "Rescuers and Superheroes."

Pokey continues, "While they were saving us that night, I looked up and could see the kids wearing superhero mask's and had red and blue superhero capes on. They came to save us!"

"Their bravery and super powers were shining so bright that the whole sky lit up! The whole sky I tell you! The night sky was lit super bright from their super powers and radiating many beautiful colors. Those kids were incredible to see!"

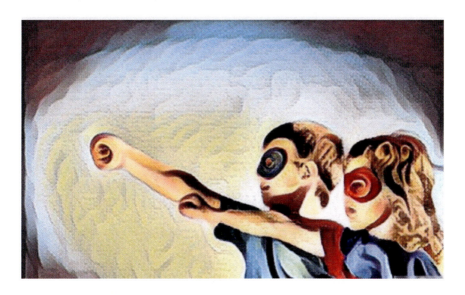

"Next, they opened our cages and took us to their truck, which had a trailer behind it. Then, they brought us here to this blessed place, the Thank you Sanctuary; where we are both safe now.

When we arrived here, the rescuers sat us down and started petting and hugging us. They told us this sanctuary is our new home, and we could live here forever!"

"What is a sanctuary?" asks Jake. Pokey explains to the kids, "A sanctuary is a place where animals are kept safe and get to enjoy their lives in peace and harmony."

"The superheroes and rescuers just want to love us, take care of us, and be our friends. They said we make them smile, laugh, and bring joy to their hearts."

"We are all very thankful because of their compassion towards animals." Rascal chimes in and asks the kids, "Do you know what compassion means?"

Nate says, "That's a big word, I'm not sure?" Rascal explains, "Well, compassion is caring about others and what happens to them."

"Yep, and since the rescuers save animals, they told us they don't eat things like bacon and ham." Says Pokey.

Jake asks, "Why is that?" Pokey points to all the pigs around the barn, and then points to himself. "Because those products are actually pig's like us."

Rascal and the kids immediately go over and give Pokey huge hugs! "It's going to get better Pokey. We will share the truth with our friends and families and we will never eat those things again. We didn't realize it was pigs like you."

Pokey says, "Great, thanks kids! You are my heroes." Now let's all get back to having fun and dancing.

Everyone walks back to the barn and continues dancing, smiling, and laughing.

Even Baby Rio is dancing in her box and twirling around. She is moving her left and right wings up and down to the beat of the music.

Rascal and the kids all hug Pokey and thank him for a fun time. Milo, (who was taking a nap,) wakes up and starts barking!

"Come on, kids! Let's go to our next adventure!" He is ready to take them to the next set of animal friends. They all begin walking down a steep hill towards some water. Is it a mirage? They hear music, and animals talking and laughing.

ADVENTURE #10. WAKEBOARDING WIGGLES, MAKING WAVES

"I saved the best for last for you kids today. Take a look at the water. See the boat cruising around?" Says Rascal. Nate squints his eyes, rubs them, then takes a second and third look. What? Wait, oh yeah, I see something!"

Rascal continues, "Now look at what is being pulled behind the boat!" The kids shout, "No way!"

"Yep, you are about to meet one of the coolest cows I know! That is the amazing, athletic, adventurous, Wiggles, the Wakeboarding Cow!" Shares Rascal.

The kids watch in awe, as wakeboarding Wiggles, (who is wearing a red life jacket and yellow helmet,) is riding waves behind the boat. She is jumping the waves the boat is creating.

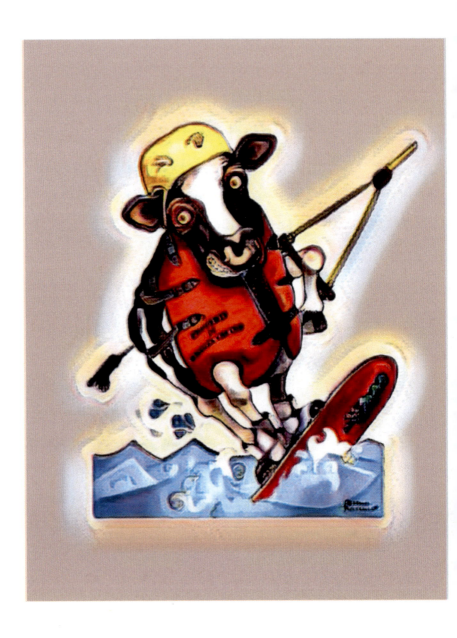

Milo tells the kids how much Wiggles loves to wakeboard. "Yep, you are right, Milo. Wiggles is a young cow that was rescued last year. Once she got to the sanctuary, she just took right to wakeboarding. She went from no smiles to a ton of smiles." Shares Rascal.

"She is incredible! She is riding the waves like a pro! Like surfers riding waves in the Hawaiian ocean," says Kaia.

Jake shouts, "Holy cow!" "That cow is awesome!" Hahaha! Everyone laughs!

Wiggles rounds the bend of the lake, jumps a wave, and releases the rope. While still on the wakeboard, she swooshes and slides all the way up to the water's edge.

Wiggles gives everyone a good soaking of water and wet splashes from the board, and the kids, Rascal, and Milo all put their hands, paws, and arms up as fast as they can to try and shield themselves from the water, but to no avail. Even Baby Rio quickly grabs the lid to her box and closes it. However, water still makes it in because Wiggles is just that good. Everyone gets soaked, but they love it!

Wiggles rides up on the sand and jumps off her board. "Hi Rascal, Hi Milo. Was that cool or what?! "Who are your wet friends?" Asks a giggling Wiggles.

"Hey kids, I'd like to introduce you to Wakeboarding Wiggles the cow." Rascal introduces everyone to Wiggles. "Nice to meet you all," I'm exhausted from all that wakeboarding. Mind if I take a break for a minute? Want to join me by the red and white, pizza shop looking picnic table over there?" Asks Wiggles.

Rascal says, "Great idea, Wiggles!" They all walk towards the picnic table and sit down. Nate wonders if he will hear some Italian music and have some pasta soon?

Jake and Kaia fall up against a tree to hold themselves up, as they can't stop laughing and smiling about what they'd just seen!

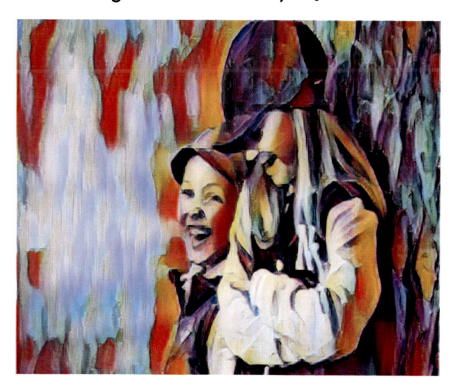

A cow, on the lake, wakeboarding behind a boat! Not to mention she was really, really good at it. She even blasted everyone with a spray of water.

Jake is laughing so hard, he accidentally snorts. That, of course, makes Kaia laugh even more!

After 15 minutes of non-stop laughter, Jake and Kaia compose themselves and walk over to the bench to join Wiggles and the group.

Kaia immediately asks Wiggles, "How did you get to the sanctuary and when did you learn to wakeboard?"

Wiggles says, "I got here a few years ago. I was rescued from a dairy farm, where they use machines to milk our mommies every day for milk and cheese. Our mommies are put in confined cages, where they can't move and have no way to escape.

When I was rescued from that farm, I knew I needed to be free, and the water became my freedom and safe place. I saw the boats on the water, picked up a wakeboard, and away I went.

At first, I was slowly and cautiously hopping over the wave wakes. Then eventually, I got braver and better and started jumping the wakes and doing tricks. I practice a lot! I really love it here and love wakeboarding out on the water!"

Wiggles continues, "I was fortunate to be rescued, but I had a difficult upbringing. My mommy and friend's mommies were all taken away from us, shortly after we were born. Imagine if you were taken away from your mommies right after your birth. Not being able to be by your mommy's side for protection, milk, and comfort?

Kaia's eyes start watering up. "That's sad, Wiggles. I'm so sorry to hear that."

Wiggles appreciates Kaia's kind words and says, "I can tell you understand. That's why you and your friends are so important to animals.

You are the generation that can save us animals, because you know the truth and have super powers to save us."

"Did you know that people eat cows?" Asks Wiggles. Nate raises his eyebrow and asks, "People eat cows like you, Wiggles?" "Why?"

"Unfortunately, yes. Hamburgers and steaks are really cow's like me that were once living?" Shares Wiggles.

"But why?" Asks Nate again. Wiggles answers, "I'm not sure why, but thankfully, some really incredible parents and kids are starting to change that.

There are tons of plant-based hamburgers now that are made without animals. This way, you can have the same taste, just minus me." Shares Wiggles.

"It's the same thing with milk. There is now Plant-Based Almond, Soy, and Cashew milk (and even chocolate milk) that tastes great and doesn't come from cows. This is helping to save us cows!

Jake say's "I'm going to ask my parents for the non-cow milk from now on."

Kaia and Nate chime in, "You got it, Wiggles. We won't drink cow's milk either."

Wiggles thanks the kids and gets up. "Hey, come join me on the boat!" Would you kids like to wakeboard? Come on, I'll show you how!"

Kids shout, "Yes! Awesome, that sounds great!" They begin walking towards the lake. Wiggles points to the wakeboard gear area and tells the kids to go inside and pick out what they want.

The kids choose their gear and jump in the boat, which has wakeboards in all different shapes, styles, and colors. There is even a sound system on the boat with two big red speakers, playing loud happy music they can hear while wakeboarding.

Wiggles takes turns teaching the kids how to wakeboard. Everyone is having a great time enjoying the sun and water!

Rascal sits in a lounge chair at the water's edge, and Baby Rio is out of her box and snuggled up closely to Rascal and Milo. They are enjoying watching Wiggles and the kid's wakeboarding on the water.

Kaia goes up first and immediately is able to ride the wake. Jake goes up next and begins riding the wakes too. Naturally, he starts goofing around and decides to let go of the rope. "Look, no hands!" Then "splash!" He falls into the water. The boat circles back around to get Jake, and he is totally fine and laughing hysterically!

Nate and the other kids decide to give it a whirl too, but they choose to ride a surfboard from behind the boat. They all nail it and ride the waves.

Wiggles plays the sounds of surf tunes for everyone's rides. After many hours of wakeboarding, Wiggles and the kids finish up and dock the boat.

Rascal thanks Wiggles for spending time with the kids, sharing her rescue story, and teaching the kids how to wakeboard and surf behind the boat.

"Please come back soon and visit us again." Says Wiggles. Everyone smiles, hugs, and departs the lake.

But as they are leaving, Nate's left eyebrow begins to slowly rise again, and he asks Rascal a question.

ADVENTURE #11. RASCAL'S RIVETING EMERGENCY RESCUE STORY

"Hey Rascal, my Uncle never did tell me how you got here. Will you tell us your story?"

"Aww... sure Nate, that is very kind of you to ask. Well, I was rescued from a small farm where I used to live."

"One day, a very fast and scary fire broke out. The fire had high flames and tons of smoke, and it was quickly burning up everything in sight."

"While in the stall with my baby brother, we could see the flames rising and the ashes falling from the sky."

"There was a thick, billowing smoke filling the air quickly. The smoke was making it difficult to breathe and we were scared because it was all happening so fast." Shared Rascal.

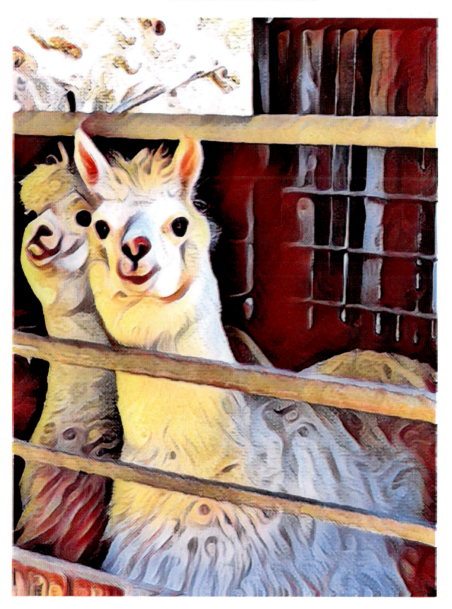

Me (Rascal) and my baby brother.

"Then, I saw some people coming towards me and I said, "Thank God!" because the fire was getting worse and we were frightened."

"As the people were opening up the gate to our stall, they brought us over to a white truck with the words "Fitzpatrick Emergency Animal Rescue" on it.

With us animals, even while someone is saving us, we are still frightened and need a little reassurance.

Outside of the Thank You, Sanctuary, you can't understand us, and we can't understand you. We just go with a hope and a prayer, a vibe and a feeling- hoping it will all be ok.

Oh yeah, and us Alpacas will lay down on the ground when we get scared, and that makes it difficult to quickly move us to safety.

We lay down and won't budge when we are scares and sometimes it makes people laugh because they can't believe we would stop and lay down during an emergency!

But we are just scared. It's always funny afterwards!" Shares Rascal.

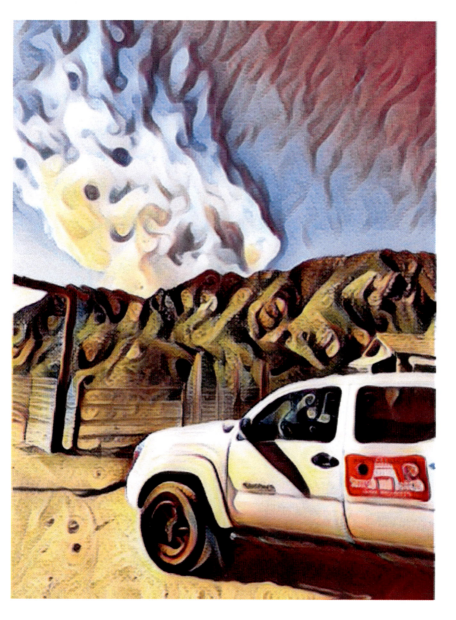

Emergency Animal Search & Rescue Truck

"When we were being rescued, there were adults and kids wearing capes, masks, and coming toward us. They were coming to save my baby brother and me!

They pulled up their truck close to us and guided us into their large, silver trailer. They were saving us and many other animals that day.

Check out this picture of me during our rescue! It wasn't very funny at the time, but I find it is hilarious now!

That's me inside the trailer, looking out the window at my new friends, the animal rescuers and superheroes. Can y'all see me in the window?

I even marked the photo with an arrow pointing towards the window, so you can't miss me." Laughed Rascal.

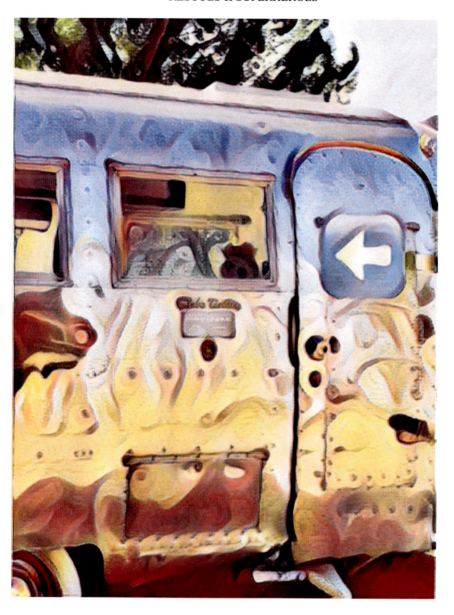

Me (Rascal) Look inside the window

Nate says, "Yes Rascal, I can see you in the window. That's a hilarious photo, and wow, what an amazing rescue story!

"Yep, I was saved from the fires and those superhero kids and family brought me here, to the Thank You, Sanctuary." Shares Rascal.

Rascal reminds the kids of the stories they heard today and how much animals are depending upon them to help rescue and save them.

"You see, us four-legged animals are kids just like you. We have mommies, daddies, and brothers and sisters too. We feel joy and sorrow, love and pain, happiness and sadness, hunger and thirst. We have feelings, just... like... you!

Now you get to use your superpowers when you protect us. I promise it will make you feel really happy and special!" Says Rascal.

ADVENTURE #12. SUPERHERO POWERS YOU'LL ALWAYS HAVE

"Because of the kindness you showed us animals today and your commitment to protecting animals, you will find a very special teddy bear with your name on it.

These are our special gifts to you and a reminder that animals need you. We can't speak in the real world and we can't protect ourselves without you." Shares Rascal.

The kids all exclaim at once, "Thank you so much!" Hugs are shared, and the kids say their goodbyes. The school bus has returned and is out front to pick them up.

As they are heading to the school bus, all of the kids find teddy bears with their names on them. The kids shout, "Thank You!"

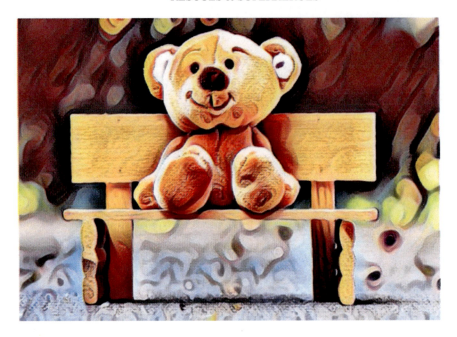

Then a whisper is heard in the distance. A peep of a sound which is very faint and not loud enough to make out what is being said.

Then the sound grows louder, and the kids look down and see Baby Rio jumping out of her box.

Baby Rio is shouting, (with her new-found voice of strength and confidence,) "Thank You!

Baby Rio is out of her box, standing tall and confident, and say's with pure happiness and joy, "Thank you!" "You showed me love, kindness, and protection today and I will never forget you.

Baby Rio continues, "With kids like you, I'm confident that animals have a new voice, a new set of protectors and superheroes- and that's you!"

"THANK YOU!"

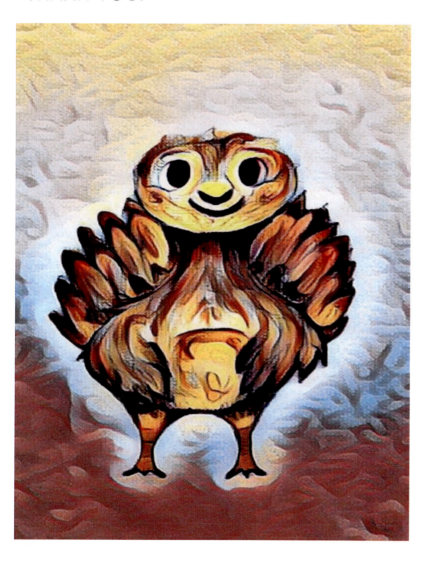

All of a sudden, Kaia shouts out, "Jake, look at your back! You have a cape! And your face, it has a mask on it! You got your super-powers!"

Jake quickly turns around and says, "I do?" "WOW!" Jake says, "Kaia, you Nate and the other kids do too!

And the kids earned their super powers that day and promised to use them always. They are super-heroes now, with super-powers to always protect animals.

And the kids shouted once more with much enthusiasm, "THANK YOU!"

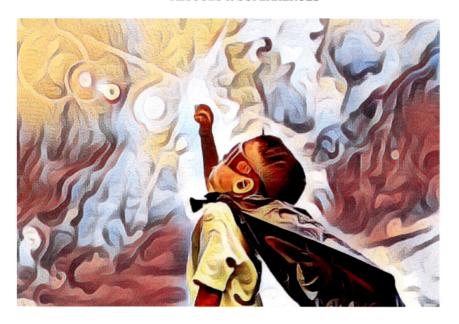

As the kids approach the school bus doors, Nate waves goodbye and walks back to the main house with Rascal and Milo.

When unexpectantly, a small, furry, animal runs past them yelling, "Quick, I need your help!" Nate smiles and says, "You've got it, we will help you. We are Superheroes now!"

And off they go to their new rescue adventure!

To the readers of our story:

Will you earn your super powers?

Will you promise to protect animals, love animals, and not eat them?

Yes? Yes! Really? Awesome!

Great! Thank you!

And all the animals of the world thank you!

XO

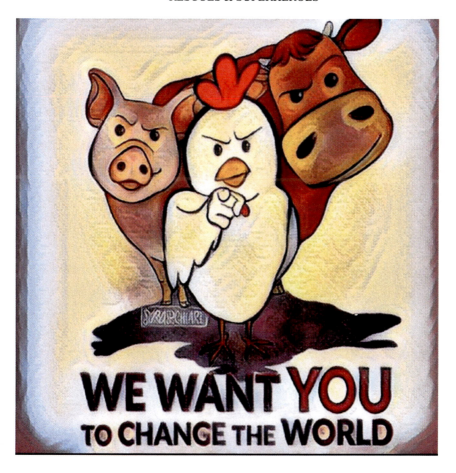

Credits:

Illustrations by leading artist: **J.B. Mann.** Wiggles the Wakeboarding Cow, Chilli the Chicken, and Pokey the Pig. @Facebook Fuzzballs*Fuzzywinks Illustrations

Illustration by: Animal Rights Artist, **Sara Sechi** - "We Want You To Change The World" @SaraSechiArt.bigcartel.com

Illustration by: **Addy Rivera Sonda.** "Put animals in your heart, Not in your belly" by leading artist, Instagram @Addy_Rivera

Illustrations by: 13 yr old, up and coming artist, **Isabelle Sebourn** - Baby Rio.

Pictures by: **Fitzpatrick Rescue** -Rascal and baby brother during the rescue, Rascal in trailer, rescue truck, AJ, Milo and Bobo.

Picture enhancements by: **Shelley Savoy@** smsavoycoverdesigns@gmail.com

About the author: Shelly Fitzpatrick

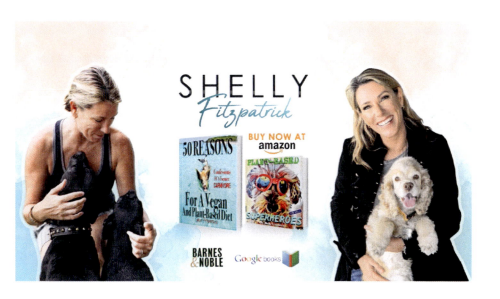

Shelly Fitzpatrick is also the author of "50 Reasons for a Vegan and Plant-Based Diet" book. She wrote this book to provide 50 great reasons to make positive changes for animals, the environment, and personal health.

Her passion is helping animals, teaching people about plant-based and dairy-free options, and fighting against the dog meat trade in South Korea and Asia.

You can get your copy at Barnes and Noble, iTunes, Google Books, and Amazon. This book is great for people 16+ and gives you...

50 Reasons for a Vegan and Plant-Based diet.

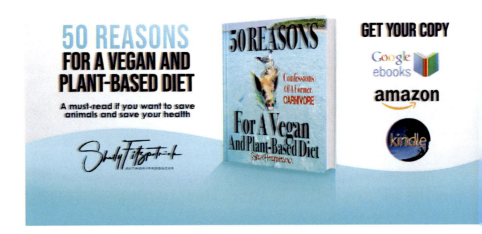

*Purchases of these books will help us to donate books to youth centers, hospitals, and charities.

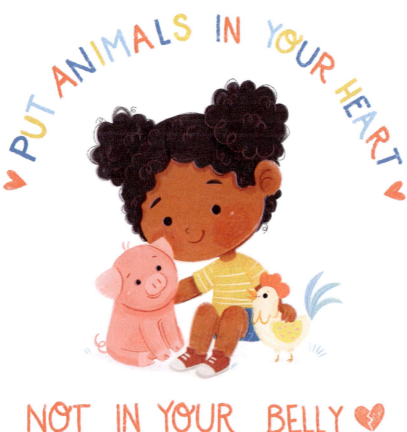

Made in the USA
Las Vegas, NV
15 December 2021